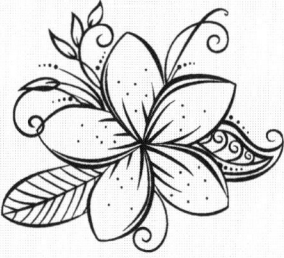

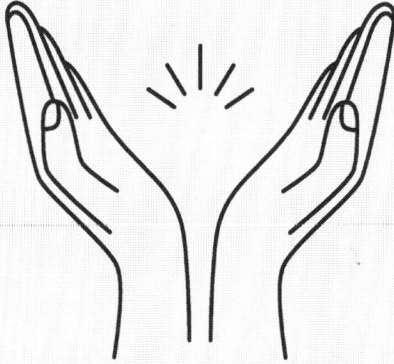

THIS GRATITUDE JOURNAL
BELONGS TO

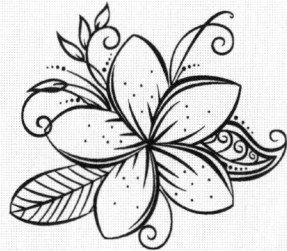

THANK YOU

Hello,

Thank you for choosing this gratitude journal as your companion on a journey that's deeply personal and enriching. Your decision to focus on gratitude every day is a powerful step towards a life filled with more joy and appreciation.

This journal is your private sanctuary for thoughts, a quiet corner for reflection, and a daily reminder of the beauty in the world around you. Each entry you make is a celebration of the good in your life, both big and small.

Remember, your journey is unique and your experiences are valuable. If you ever wish to share your stories of gratitude or have thoughts to express, I'm here to listen. You can reach out to me at:

Website: www.rblwellnessbeauty.com
Email: info@rblwellnessbeauty.com or redesignbuildlive@gmail.com

Thank you for inviting this journal into your daily routine. May it be a source of joy and a reflection of the wonderful things in your life.

With heartfelt thanks,

Allison Woodley-Tyehimba.
Founder of RBL Wellness & Beauty

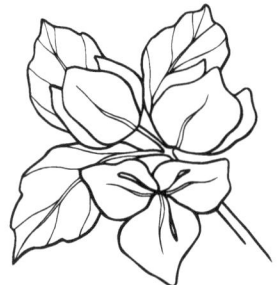

"When gratitude becomes an essential foundation in our lives, miracles start to appear everywhere." - Emmanuel Dagher

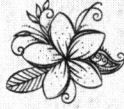

Day/Date: _____

Today I am Grateful for _____

_____

_____

_____

Day/Date: _____

Today I am Grateful for: _____

_____

_____

_____

"To be grateful is to find blessings in everything, even the smallest of things."

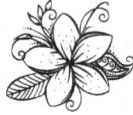

Day/Date: _____

Today I am Grateful for _____

_____

_____

_____

Day/Date: _____

Today I am Grateful for: _____

_____

_____

_____

"The beauty of life blooms from a garden of gratitude."

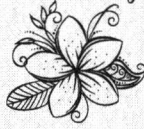

Day/Date: _____

Today I am Grateful for _____

_____

_____

_____

Day/Date: _____

Today I am Grateful for: _____

_____

_____

_____

5

"Embrace your journey with thanks: every step has its own magic."

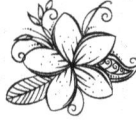

Day/Date: _____

Today I am Grateful for _____

_____

_____

_____

Day/Date: _____

Today I am Grateful for: _____

_____

_____

_____

"Thankfulness is the soil in which joy thrives."

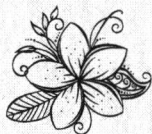

Day/Date: _____

Today I am Grateful for _____

_____

_____

_____

Day/Date: _____

Today I am Grateful for: _____

_____

_____

_____

6

"Gratitude turns what we have into enough, and more."

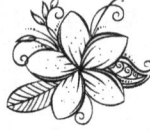

Day/Date: _____

Today I am Grateful for _____

_____

_____

_____

Day/Date: _____

Today I am Grateful for: _____

_____

_____

_____

"Count blessings, not burdens; seek beauty, not flaws."

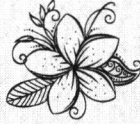

Day/Date: _____

Today I am Grateful for _____

_____

_____

_____

Day/Date: _____

Today I am Grateful for: _____

_____

_____

_____

"In the quiet moments, find gratitude for the unsung melodies of life."

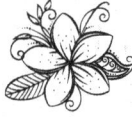

Day/Date: _____

Today I am Grateful for _____

_____

_____

_____

Day/Date: _____

Today I am Grateful for: _____

_____

_____

_____

"Gratitude is the song of the soul, sung in harmony with life's journey."

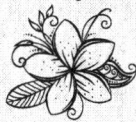

Day/Date: _____

Today I am Grateful for _____

_____

_____

_____

Day/Date: _____

Today I am Grateful for: _____

_____

_____

_____

"Celebrate yourself; every milestone, big or small, is a victory of spirit."

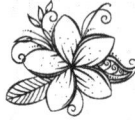

Day/Date: _____

Today I am Grateful for _____

_____

_____

_____

Day/Date: _____

Today I am Grateful for: _____

_____

_____

_____

"With a grateful heart, every experience is a lesson and a blessing."

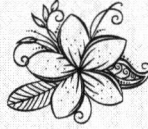

Day/Date: _____

Today I am Grateful for _____

_____

_____

_____

Day/Date: _____

Today I am Grateful for: _____

_____

_____

_____

"Let gratitude be your compass and joy your path."

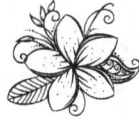

Day/Date: _____

Today I am Grateful for _____

_____

_____

_____

Day/Date: _____

Today I am Grateful for: _____

_____

_____

_____

"Gratitude is an art of painting an adversity into a lovely picture." - Kak Sri

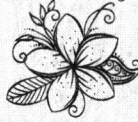

Day/Date: _____

Today I am Grateful for _____

_____

_____

_____

Day/Date: _____

Today I am Grateful for: _____

_____

_____

_____

"Gratitude is the open door to abundance."

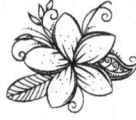

Day/Date: _____

Today I am Grateful for _____

_____

_____

_____

Day/Date: _____

Today I am Grateful for: _____

_____

_____

_____

"Gratitude is the memory of the heart." - Jean Baptiste Massieu

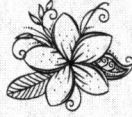

Day/Date: _____

Today I am Grateful for _____

_____

_____

_____

Day/Date: _____

Today I am Grateful for: _____

_____

_____

_____

"When you are grateful, fear disappears and abundance appears." - Tony Robbins.

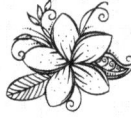

Day/Date: _____

Today I am Grateful for _____

_____

_____

_____

Day/Date: _____

Today I am Grateful for: _____

_____

_____

_____

"The thankful receiver bears a plentiful harvest." – William Blake.

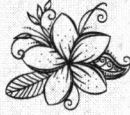

Day/Date: _____

Today I am Grateful for _____

_____

_____

_____

Day/Date: _____

Today I am Grateful for: _____

_____

_____

_____

"Gratitude is not in the words but in the heart which expresses it.
Luffina Lourduraj

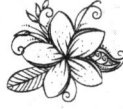

Day/Date: _____

Today I am Grateful for _____

_____

_____

_____

Day/Date: _____

Today I am Grateful for: _____

_____

_____

_____

"Gratitude is the vitamin for the soul."

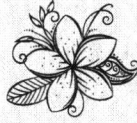

Day/Date: _____

Today I am Grateful for _____

_____

_____

_____

Day/Date: _____

Today I am Grateful for: _____

_____

_____

_____

"Gratitude is the seed of gladness."

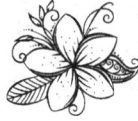

Day/Date: _____

Today I am Grateful for _____

_____

_____

_____

Day/Date: _____

Today I am Grateful for: _____

_____

_____

_____

"Gratitude transforms the torment of memory into silent joy."

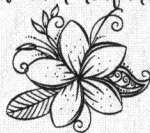

Day/Date: _____

Today I am Grateful for _____

_____

_____

_____

Day/Date: _____

Today I am Grateful for: _____

_____

_____

_____

"Gratitude is the echo of kindness in the heart."

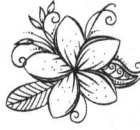

Day/Date: _____

Today I am Grateful for _____

_____

_____

_____

Day/Date: _____

Today I am Grateful for: _____

_____

_____

_____

"Embrace gratitude as a lifestyle, not just a moment."

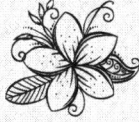

Day/Date: _____

Today I am Grateful for _____

_____

_____

_____

Day/Date: _____

Today I am Grateful for: _____

_____

_____

_____

"Every moment of gratitude makes a difference in your attitude." - Bruce Wilkinson

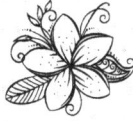

Day/Date: _____

Today I am Grateful for _____

_____

_____

_____

Day/Date: _____

Today I am Grateful for: _____

_____

_____

_____

"Gratitude is the music of the soul's deepest harmony."

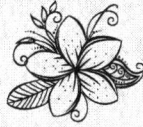

Day/Date: _____

Today I am Grateful for _____

_____

_____

_____

Day/Date: _____

Today I am Grateful for: _____

_____

_____

_____

"A grateful heart is a magnet for miracles."

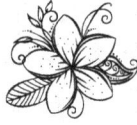

Day/Date: _____

Today I am Grateful for _____

_____

_____

_____

Day/Date: _____

Today I am Grateful for: _____

_____

_____

_____

"Gratitude creates a vision of abundance, painting our experiences with vibrant colors of hope."

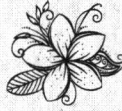

Day/Date: _____

Today I am Grateful for _____

_____

_____

_____

Day/Date: _____

Today I am Grateful for: _____

_____

_____

_____

"Gratitude turns ordinary opportunities into blessings."
William Arthur War

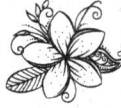

Day/Date: _____

Today I am Grateful for _____

_____

_____

_____

Day/Date: _____

Today I am Grateful for: _____

_____

_____

_____

"The attitude of gratitude brings opportunities."

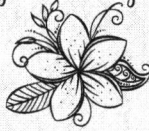

Day/Date: _____

Today I am Grateful for _____

_____

_____

_____

Day/Date: _____

Today I am Grateful for: _____

_____

_____

_____

"Gratitude is the light that opens the soul to its essence." - Unknown

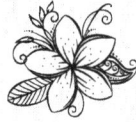

Day/Date: _____

Today I am Grateful for _____

_____

_____

_____

Day/Date: _____

Today I am Grateful for: _____

_____

_____

_____

"Gratitude is the fairest blossom which springs from the soul."
Henry Ward Beecher

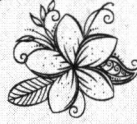

Day/Date: _____

Today I am Grateful for _____

_____

_____

_____

Day/Date: _____

Today I am Grateful for: _____

_____

_____

_____

"A life filled with gratitude is a life filled with joy."

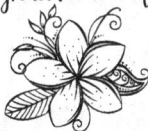

Day/Date: _____

Today I am Grateful for _____

_____

_____

_____

Day/Date: _____

Today I am Grateful for: _____

_____

_____

_____

"Gratitude is the fairest blossom which springs from the soul."
Henry Ward Beecher

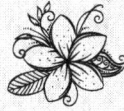

Day/Date: _____

Today I am Grateful for _____

_____

_____

_____

Day/Date: _____

Today I am Grateful for: _____

_____

_____

_____

"Gratitude is the fairest blossom which springs from the soul."
Henry Ward Beecher

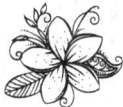

Day/Date: _____

Today I am Grateful for _____

_____

_____

_____

Day/Date: _____

Today I am Grateful for: _____

_____

_____

_____

"Gratitude turns what we have into enough, and more."
Melody Beattie.

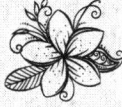

Day/Date: _____

Today I am Grateful for _____

_____

_____

_____

Day/Date: _____

Today I am Grateful for: _____

_____

_____

_____

"Gratitude and attitude are not challenges: they are choices." -Robert Braathe

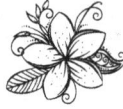

Day/Date: _____

Today I am Grateful for _____

_____

_____

_____

Day/Date: _____

Today I am Grateful for: _____

_____

_____

_____

"Gratitude is the most exquisite form of courtesy." - Jacques Maritain

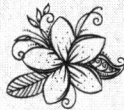

Day/Date: _____

Today I am Grateful for _____

_____

_____

_____

Day/Date: _____

Today I am Grateful for: _____

_____

_____

_____

"Gratitude is the heart's memory." - French Proverb

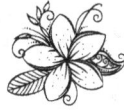

Day/Date: _____

Today I am Grateful for _____

_____

_____

_____

Day/Date: _____

Today I am Grateful for: _____

_____

_____

_____

"Gratitude is the most beautiful way to remember our blessings."

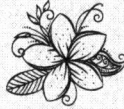

Day/Date: _____

Today I am Grateful for _____

_____

_____

_____

Day/Date: _____

Today I am Grateful for: _____

_____

_____

_____

"Gratitude is a powerful catalyst for happiness." -Amy Colletter

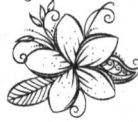

Day/Date: _____

Today I am Grateful for _____

_____

_____

_____

Day/Date: _____

Today I am Grateful for: _____

_____

_____

_____

"Gratitude is the sweetest thing in a seeker's life in all human life." - Sri Chinmoy

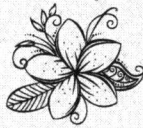

Day/Date: _____

Today I am Grateful for _____

_____

_____

_____

Day/Date: _____

Today I am Grateful for: _____

_____

_____

_____

"The essence of all beautiful art, all great art, is gratitude."
Friedrich Nietzsche

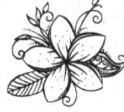

Day/Date: _____

Today I am Grateful for _____

_____

_____

_____

Day/Date: _____

Today I am Grateful for: _____

_____

_____

_____

"Train yourself never to put off the word or action for the expression of gratitude."
Albert Schweitzer

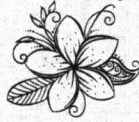

Day/Date: _____

Today I am Grateful for _____

_____

_____

_____

Day/Date: _____

Today I am Grateful for: _____

_____

_____

_____

"Gratitude is not only the greatest of virtues but the parent of all others." - Cicero.

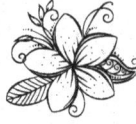

Day/Date: _____

Today I am Grateful for _____

_____

_____

_____

Day/Date: _____

Today I am Grateful for: _____

_____

_____

_____

"Act with kindness, but do not expect gratitude." - Confucius

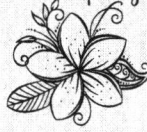

Day/Date: _____

Today I am Grateful for _____

_____

_____

_____

Day/Date: _____

Today I am Grateful for: _____

_____

_____

_____

Gratitude Reflections

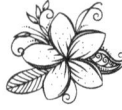

Looking back over the past three months, what changes have you noticed in your attitude towards yourself and others as a result of maintaining a gratitude journal?

How has this practice influenced your daily life, relationships, and overall well-being?"

"If the only prayer you said in your whole life was, 'thank you,' that would suffice."
Meister Eckhart.

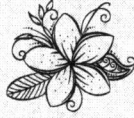

Day/Date: _____

Today I am Grateful for _____

_____

_____

_____

Day/Date: _____

Today I am Grateful for: _____

_____

_____

_____

"The deepest craving of human nature is the need to be appreciated."
William James

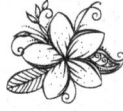

Day/Date: _____

Today I am Grateful for _____

_____

_____

_____

Day/Date: _____

Today I am Grateful for: _____

_____

_____

_____

"Gratitude is the memory of the heart." – Jean Baptiste Massieu

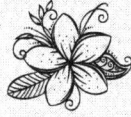

Day/Date: _____

Today I am Grateful for _____

_____

_____

_____

Day/Date: _____

Today I am Grateful for: _____

_____

_____

_____

"Gratitude looks to the past and love to the present: fear, avarice, lust, and ambition look ahead." - C.S. Lewis

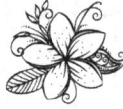

Day/Date: _____

Today I am Grateful for _____

_____

_____

_____

Day/Date: _____

Today I am Grateful for: _____

_____

_____

_____

"Gratitude can transform common days into thanksgivings."
William Arthur Ward

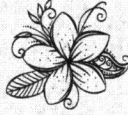

Day/Date: _____

Today I am Grateful for _____

_____

_____

_____

Day/Date: _____

Today I am Grateful for: _____

_____

_____

_____

"Joy is the simplest form of gratitude." ~ Karl Barth

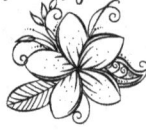

Day/Date: _____

Today I am Grateful for _____

_____

_____

_____

Day/Date: _____

Today I am Grateful for: _____

_____

_____

_____

"Gratitude turns what we have into enough."

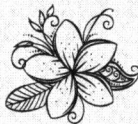

Day/Date: _____

Today I am Grateful for _____

_____

_____

_____

Day/Date: _____

Today I am Grateful for: _____

_____

_____

_____

"Gratitude is the healthiest of all human emotions." - Zig Ziglar

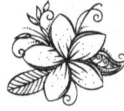

Day/Date: _____

Today I am Grateful for _____

_____

_____

_____

Day/Date: _____

Today I am Grateful for: _____

_____

_____

_____

"Wear gratitude like a cloak, and it will feed every corner of your life." -Rumi

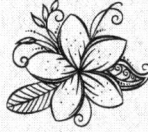

Day/Date: _____

"Today I am Grateful for_____

_____

_____

_____

Day/Date: _____

Today I am Grateful for:_____

_____

_____

_____

"Gratitude is the wine for the soul. Go on. Get drunk." - Rumi.

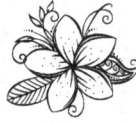

Day/Date: _____

Today I am Grateful for _____

_____

_____

_____

Day/Date: _____

Today I am Grateful for: _____

_____

_____

_____

"The more grateful I am, the more beauty I see." - Mary Davis

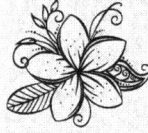

Day/Date: _____

Today I am Grateful for _____

_____

_____

_____

Day/Date: _____

Today I am Grateful for: _____

_____

_____

_____

``Gratitude is a powerful catalyst for happiness.`` - Amy Collette.

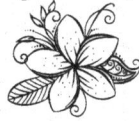

Day/Date: _____

Today I am Grateful for _____

_____

_____

_____

Day/Date: _____

Today I am Grateful for: _____

_____

_____

_____

"Gratitude is the sign of noble souls." - Aesop

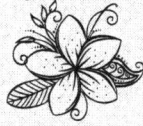

Day/Date: _____

Today I am Grateful for _____

_____

_____

_____

Day/Date: _____

Today I am Grateful for: _____

_____

_____

_____

"Gratitude makes what we have enough."

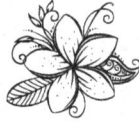

Day/Date: _____

Today I am Grateful for _____

_____

_____

_____

Day/Date: _____

Today I am Grateful for: _____

_____

_____

_____

"Act with kindness, but do not expect gratitude." - Confucius.

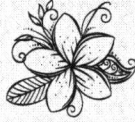

Day/Date: _____

Today I am Grateful for _____

_____

_____

_____

Day/Date: _____

Today I am Grateful for: _____

_____

_____

_____

"The deepest craving of human nature is the need to be appreciated."
William James

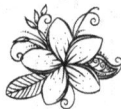

Day/Date: _____

Today I am Grateful for _____

_____

_____

_____

Day/Date: _____

Today I am Grateful for: _____

_____

_____

_____

"Gratitude is the fairest blossom which springs from the soul."
Henry Ward Beecher.

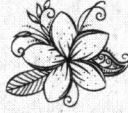

Day/Date: _____

Today I am Grateful for _____

_____

_____

_____

Day/Date: _____

Today I am Grateful for: _____

_____

_____

_____

"Gratitude is not only the greatest of virtues but the parent of all others." - Cicero.

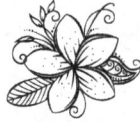

Day/Date: _____

Today I am Grateful for _____

_____

_____

_____

Day/Date: _____

Today I am Grateful for: _____

_____

_____

_____

"Gratitude is the most beautiful way to remember our blessings."

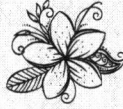

Day/Date: _____

Today I am Grateful for _____

_____

_____

_____

Day/Date: _____

Today I am Grateful for: _____

_____

_____

_____

"Gratitude is the heart's memory." – French Proverb

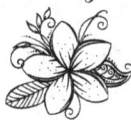

Day/Date: _____

Today I am Grateful for _____

_____

_____

_____

Day/Date: _____

Today I am Grateful for: _____

_____

_____

_____

"Living in a state of gratitude is the gateway to grace." - Arianna Huffington

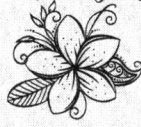

Day/Date: _____

Today I am Grateful for _____

_____

_____

_____

Day/Date: _____

Today I am Grateful for: _____

_____

_____

_____

"Gratitude is riches. Complaint is poverty." - Doris Day

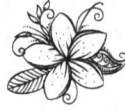

Day/Date: _____

Today I am Grateful for _____

_____

_____

_____

Day/Date: _____

Today I am Grateful for: _____

_____

_____

_____

"If you want to turn your life around, try thankfulness.
It will change your life mightily." - Gerald Good

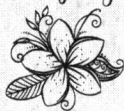

Day/Date: _____

Today I am Grateful for _____

_____

_____

_____

Day/Date: _____

Today I am Grateful for: _____

_____

_____

_____

"Gratitude is riches. Complaint is poverty." - Doris Day.

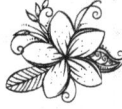

Day/Date: _____

Today I am Grateful for _____

_____

_____

_____

Day/Date: _____

Today I am Grateful for: _____

_____

_____

_____

"Appreciation is a wonderful thing. It makes what is excellent in others belong to us as well." -Voltaire.

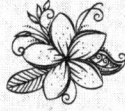

Day/Date: _____

Today I am Grateful for _____

_____

_____

_____

Day/Date: _____

Today I am Grateful for: _____

_____

_____

_____

"Be thankful for what you have; you'll end up having more." - Oprah Winfrey

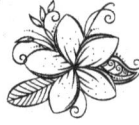

Day/Date: _____

Today I am Grateful for _____

_____

_____

_____

Day/Date: _____

Today I am Grateful for: _____

_____

_____

_____

"Gratitude is the sweetest thing in a seeker's life in all human life." - Sri Chinmoy

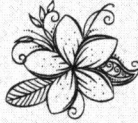

Day/Date: _____

Today I am Grateful for _____

_____

_____

_____

Day/Date: _____

Today I am Grateful for: _____

_____

_____

_____

"Gratitude is a powerful catalyst for happiness." - Amy Collette

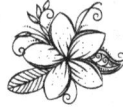

Day/Date: _____

Today I am Grateful for _____

_____

_____

_____

Day/Date: _____

Today I am Grateful for: _____

_____

_____

_____

"Gratitude is the open door to abundance."

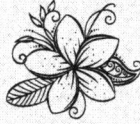

Day/Date: _____

Today I am Grateful for _____

_____

_____

_____

Day/Date: _____

Today I am Grateful for: _____

_____

_____

_____

"Gratitude is the wine for the soul. Go on. Get drunk." - Rumi

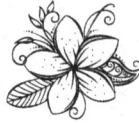

Day/Date: _____

Today I am Grateful for _____

_____

_____

_____

Day/Date: _____

Today I am Grateful for: _____

_____

_____

_____

"The only people with whom you should try to get even are those who have helped you"
John E. Southard

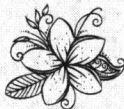

Day/Date: _____

Today I am Grateful for _____

_____

_____

_____

Day/Date: _____

Today I am Grateful for: _____

_____

_____

_____

"You are the captain of your soul; steer it towards your dreams"

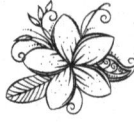

Day/Date: _____

Today I am Grateful for _____

_____

_____

_____

Day/Date: _____

Today I am Grateful for: _____

_____

_____

_____

"Gratitude is the most exquisite form of courtesy." - Jacques Maritain.

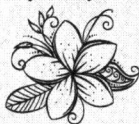

Day/Date: _____

Today I am Grateful for _____

_____

_____

_____

Day/Date: _____

Today I am Grateful for: _____

_____

_____

_____

"When I started counting my blessings, my whole life turned around."
Willie Nelson.

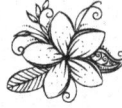

Day/Date: _____

Today I am Grateful for _____

_____

_____

_____

Day/Date: _____

Today I am Grateful for: _____

_____

_____

_____

"Gratitude paints little smiley faces on everything it touches."
Richelle E. Goodrich.

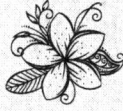

Day/Date: _____

Today I am Grateful for _____

_____

_____

_____

Day/Date: _____

Today I am Grateful for: _____

_____

_____

_____

"The root of joy is gratefulness." - David Steindl-Rast

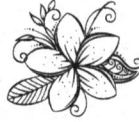

Day/Date: _____

Today I am Grateful for _____

_____

_____

_____

Day/Date: _____

Today I am Grateful for: _____

_____

_____

_____

"Gratitude can transform common days into thanksgivings."
William Arthur Ward.

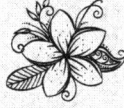

Day/Date: _____

Today I am Grateful for _____

_____

_____

_____

Day/Date: _____

Today I am Grateful for: _____

_____

_____

_____

"You are the captain of your soul; steer it towards your dreams".

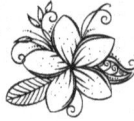

Day/Date: _____

Today I am Grateful for _____

_____

_____

_____

Day/Date: _____

Today I am Grateful for: _____

_____

_____

_____

"Gratitude turns what we have into enough."

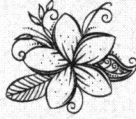

Day/Date: _____

*Today I am Grateful for*_____

_____

_____

_____

Day/Date: _____

*Today I am Grateful for:*_____

_____

_____

_____

"Gratitude makes sense of our past, brings peace for today, and creates a vision for tomorrow." - Melody Beattie.

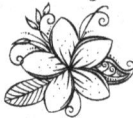

Day/Date: _____

Today I am Grateful for _____

_____

_____

_____

Day/Date: _____

Today I am Grateful for: _____

_____

_____

_____

"Gratitude is the healthiest of all human emotions." - Zig Ziglar

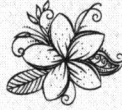

Day/Date: _____

Today I am Grateful for _____

_____

_____

_____

Day/Date: _____

Today I am Grateful for: _____

_____

_____

_____

"Gratitude is the sign of noble souls." -Aesop.

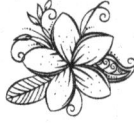

Day/Date: _____

Today I am Grateful for _____

_____

_____

_____

Day/Date: _____

Today I am Grateful for: _____

_____

_____

_____

"Gratitude is the memory of the heart." - Jean Baptiste Massieu

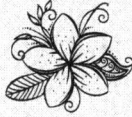

Day/Date: _____

Today I am Grateful for _____

_____

_____

_____

Day/Date: _____

Today I am Grateful for: _____

_____

_____

_____

"Silent gratitude isn't very much to anyone." - Gertrude Stein.

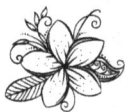

Day/Date: _____

Today I am Grateful for _____

_____

_____

_____

Day/Date: _____

Today I am Grateful for: _____

_____

_____

_____

"Silent gratitude isn't very much to anyone." _ Gertrude Stein.

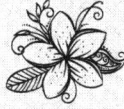

Day/Date: _____

Today I am Grateful for _____

_____

_____

_____

Day/Date: _____

Today I am Grateful for: _____

_____

_____

_____

Gratitude Reflection

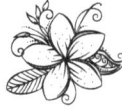

How has my perspective on life changed since starting this gratitude journal?

Are there specific moments or events where I felt a stronger sense of gratitude than usual?

"Gratitude is the fairest blossom which springs from the soul."
Henry Ward Beecher

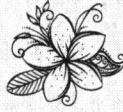

Day/Date: _____

Today I am Grateful for _____

_____

_____

_____

Day/Date: _____

Today I am Grateful for: _____

_____

_____

_____

"Joy is the simplest form of gratitude." - Karl Barth

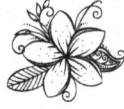

Day/Date: _____

Today I am Grateful for _____

_____

_____

_____

Day/Date: _____

Today I am Grateful for: _____

_____

_____

_____

"Gratitude is the art of painting adversity into a masterpiece of growth."

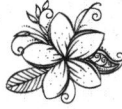

Day/Date: _____

Today I am Grateful for_____

_____

_____

_____

Day/Date: _____

Today I am Grateful for:_____

_____

_____

_____

"Gratitude is the most passionate transformative force in the cosmos."
Sarah Ban Breathnach

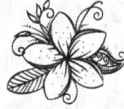

Day/Date: _____

Today I am Grateful for _____

_____

_____

_____

Day/Date: _____

Today I am Grateful for: _____

_____

_____

_____

"Gratitude is the wine for the soul. Go on. Get drunk." - Rumi

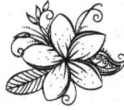

Day/Date: _____

Today I am Grateful for _____

_____

_____

Day/Date: _____

Today I am Grateful for: _____

_____

_____

"Gratitude changes the pangs of memory into a tranquil joy." - Dietrich Bonhoeffer

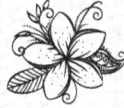

Day/Date: _____

Today I am Grateful for _____

_____

_____

_____

Day/Date: _____

Today I am Grateful for: _____

_____

_____

_____

"Gratitude is merely the secret hope of further favors."
Francois de La Rochefoucauld

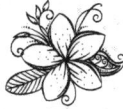

Day/Date: _____

Today I am Grateful for _____

_____

_____

_____

Day/Date: _____

Today I am Grateful for: _____

_____

_____

_____

"An attitude of gratitude brings great things." - Yogi Bhajan

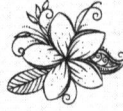

Day/Date: _____

Today I am Grateful for _____

_____

_____

_____

Day/Date: _____

Today I am Grateful for: _____

_____

_____

_____

"Gratitude is a duty which ought to be paid, but which none have a right to expect."
Jean-Jacques Rousseau

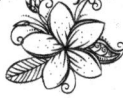

Day/Date: _____

Today I am Grateful for _____

_____

_____

_____

Day/Date: _____

Today I am Grateful for: _____

_____

_____

_____

"Train yourself never to put off the word or action for the expression of gratitude."
Albert Schweitzer.

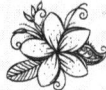

Day/Date: _____

Today I am Grateful for _____

_____

_____

_____

Day/Date: _____

Today I am Grateful for: _____

_____

_____

_____

"Be thankful for everything that happens in your life; it's all an experience."
Roy T. Bennett

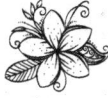

Day/Date: _____

Today I am Grateful for _____

_____

_____

_____

Day/Date: _____

Today I am Grateful for: _____

_____

_____

_____

"Gratitude is the memory of the heart." -Jean Baptiste Massieu

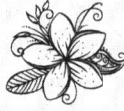

Day/Date: _____

Today I am Grateful for _____

_____

_____

_____

Day/Date: _____

Today I am Grateful for: _____

_____

_____

_____

"Gratitude is the most effective way of getting into harmony with the Universe."
Wallace Wattles

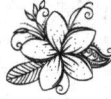

Day/Date: _____

Today I am Grateful for _____

_____

_____

_____

Day/Date: _____

Today I am Grateful for: _____

_____

_____

_____

"The only people with whom you should try to get even are those who have helped you."
John E. Southard

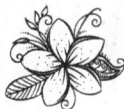

Day/Date: _____

Today I am Grateful for _____

_____

_____

_____

Day/Date: _____

Today I am Grateful for: _____

_____

_____

_____

"Wear gratitude like a cloak, and it will feed every corner of your life." - Rumi

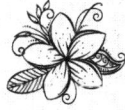

Day/Date: _____

Today I am Grateful for _____

_____

_____

_____

Day/Date: _____

Today I am Grateful for: _____

_____

_____

_____

"Gratitude is the completion of thankfulness. Thankfulness may consist merely of words. Gratitude is shown in acts." - Henri Frederic Amiel

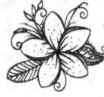

Day/Date: _____

Today I am Grateful for _____

_____

_____

_____

Day/Date: _____

Today I am Grateful for: _____

_____

_____

_____

"The more you practice the art of thankfulness, the more you have to be thankful for."
Norman Vincent Peale

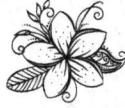

Day/Date: _____

Today I am Grateful for _____

_____

_____

_____

Day/Date: _____

Today I am Grateful for: _____

_____

_____

_____

"Gratitude is the sweetest of the heart's whispers." - Richelle E. Goodrich

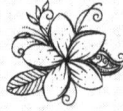

Day/Date: _____

Today I am Grateful for _____

_____

_____

Day/Date: _____

Today I am Grateful for: _____

_____

_____

"Gratitude looks to the past and love to the present: fear, avarice, lust, and ambition look ahead." - C.S. Lewis

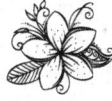

Day/Date: _____

Today I am Grateful for _____

_____

_____

_____

Day/Date: _____

Today I am Grateful for: _____

_____

_____

_____

"Gratitude is an opener of locked-up blessings." - Marianne Williamson

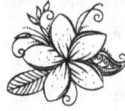

Day/Date: _____

Today I am Grateful for _____

_____

_____

_____

Day/Date: _____

Today I am Grateful for: _____

_____

_____

_____

"When gratitude becomes an essential foundation in our lives, miracles start to appear everywhere." - Emmanuel Dalgher

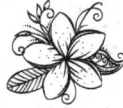

Day/Date: _____

Today I am Grateful for _____

_____

_____

_____

Day/Date: _____

Today I am Grateful for: _____

_____

_____

_____

"Gratitude is not a tool with which to fool the Mind; it is a tool that opens the Mind."
Ryan Lilly

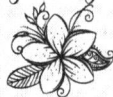

Day/Date: _____

Today I am Grateful for _____

_____

_____

_____

Day/Date: _____

Today I am Grateful for: _____

_____

_____

_____

"The struggle ends when gratitude begins." - Neale Donald Walsch

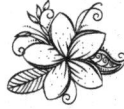

Day/Date: _____

Today I am Grateful for _____

_____

_____

_____

Day/Date: _____

Today I am Grateful for: _____

_____

_____

_____

"Gratitude is a powerful process for shifting your energy and bringing more of what you want into your life." - Rhonda Byrne

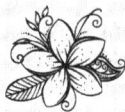

Day/Date: _____

Today I am Grateful for _____

_____

_____

_____

Day/Date: _____

Today I am Grateful for: _____

_____

_____

_____

"Gratitude doesn't change what we have; it changes how we see it." - John Maxwell

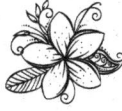

Day/Date: _____

Today I am Grateful for _____

_____

_____

_____

Day/Date: _____

Today I am Grateful for: _____

_____

_____

_____

"Gratitude is the most important key to success. It is the one key that opens all the doors to the blessings of life." -Buddha

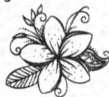

Day/Date: _____

Today I am Grateful for _____

_____

_____

_____

Day/Date: _____

Today I am Grateful for: _____

_____

_____

_____

"Gratitude is the best attitude."

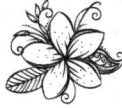

Day/Date: _____

Today I am Grateful for _____

_____

_____

_____

Day/Date: _____

Today I am Grateful for: _____

_____

_____

_____

"Gratitude is when memory is stored in the heart and not in the mind."
Lionel Hampton

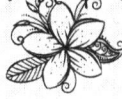

Day/Date: _____

Today I am Grateful for _____

_____

_____

_____

Day/Date: _____

Today I am Grateful for: _____

_____

_____

_____

"Gratitude is riches. Complaint is poverty." - Doris Day.

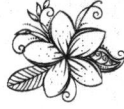

Day/Date: _____

Today I am Grateful for _____

_____

_____

_____

Day/Date: _____

Today I am Grateful for: _____

_____

_____

_____

"Gratitude is the fairest blossom which springs from the soul." -Henry Ward Beecher

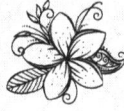

Day/Date: _____

Today I am Grateful for _____

_____

_____

_____

Day/Date: _____

Today I am Grateful for: _____

_____

_____

_____

"Gratitude is not only the memory but the homage of the heart rendered to God for His goodness." - Nathaniel Parker Willis

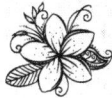

Day/Date: _____

Today I am Grateful for _____

_____

_____

_____

Day/Date: _____

Today I am Grateful for: _____

_____

_____

_____

"Gratitude is the echo of grace as it reverberates through the hollows of a human heart." - John O'Donohue

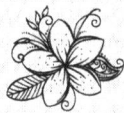

Day/Date: _____

Today I am Grateful for _____

_____

_____

_____

Day/Date: _____

Today I am Grateful for: _____

_____

_____

_____

"Thankfulness creates gratitude which generates contentment that causes peace."
Todd Stocker

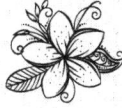

Day/Date: _____

Today I am Grateful for _____

_____

_____

_____

Day/Date: _____

Today I am Grateful for: _____

_____

_____

_____

"Gratitude is a quality similar to electricity: it must be produced and discharged and used up in order to exist at all." -William Faulkner

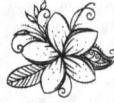

Day/Date: _____

Today I am Grateful for _____

_____

_____

_____

Day/Date: _____

Today I am Grateful for: _____

_____

_____

_____

"Practice gratitude to access joy." - Brené Brown

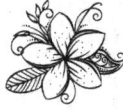

Day/Date: _____

Today I am Grateful for _____

_____

_____

_____

Day/Date: _____

Today I am Grateful for: _____

_____

_____

_____

"True gratitude comes from knowing that you belong in the infinite dance of life." -- John O'Donohue

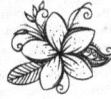

Day/Date: _____

Today I am Grateful for _____

_____

_____

_____

Day/Date: _____

Today I am Grateful for: _____

_____

_____

_____

"Give thanks for a little and you will find a lot." - Hansa Proverb.

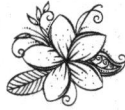

Day/Date: _____

Today I am Grateful for _____

_____

_____

_____

Day/Date: _____

Today I am Grateful for: _____

_____

_____

_____

"Gratitude is the art of painting an adversity into a lovely picture." - Kak Sri

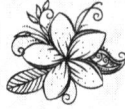

Day/Date: _____

Today I am Grateful for _____

_____

_____

_____

Day/Date: _____

Today I am Grateful for: _____

_____

_____

_____

"The heart that gives thanks is a happy one, for we cannot feel thankful and unhappy at the same time." - Douglas Wood

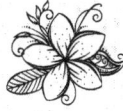

Day/Date: _____

Today I am Grateful for _____

_____

_____

_____

Day/Date: _____

Today I am Grateful for: _____

_____

_____

_____

"When we focus on our gratitude, the tide of disappointment goes out and the tide of love rushes in." - Kristin Armstrong

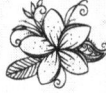

Day/Date: _____

Today I am Grateful for _____

_____

_____

_____

Day/Date: _____

Today I am Grateful for: _____

_____

_____

_____

"Silent gratitude isn't very much to anyone." - Gertrude Stein

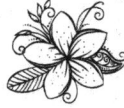

Day/Date: _____

Today I am Grateful for _____

_____

_____

_____

Day/Date: _____

Today I am Grateful for: _____

_____

_____

_____

"moment of gratitude makes a difference in your attitude." -Bruce Wilkinson

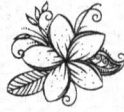

Day/Date: _____

Today I am Grateful for _____

_____

_____

_____

Day/Date: _____

Today I am Grateful for: _____

_____

_____

_____

"If you want to find happiness, find gratitude." - Steve Maraboli

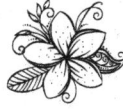

Day/Date: _____

Today I am Grateful for _____

_____

_____

_____

Day/Date: _____

Today I am Grateful for: _____

_____

_____

_____

"Acknowledging the good that you already have in your life is the foundation for all abundance." - Eckhart Tolle

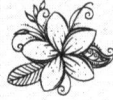

Day/Date: _____

Today I am Grateful for _____

_____

_____

_____

Day/Date: _____

Today I am Grateful for: _____

_____

_____

_____

Gratitude Reflection

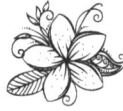

What lessons have I learned about gratitude and its impact on my life?

How have these last 90 days of gratitude affected my relationships with myself and others?

"Gratitude is merely the secret hope of further favors." - Francois de La Rochefoucauld

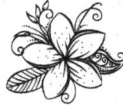

Day/Date: _____

Today I am Grateful for _____

_____

_____

_____

Day/Date: _____

Today I am Grateful for: _____

_____

_____

_____

"Gratitude is richer than regret."

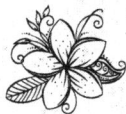

Day/Date: _____

Today I am Grateful for _____

_____

_____

_____

Day/Date: _____

Today I am Grateful for: _____

_____

_____

_____

"Gratitude is the most exquisite form of courtesy." - Jacques Maritain

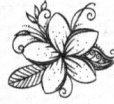

Day/Date: _____

Today I am Grateful for _____

_____

_____

_____

Day/Date: _____

Today I am Grateful for: _____

_____

_____

_____

"Gratitude is the music of the heart, when its chords are swept by the breeze of kindness." - Unknown

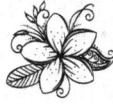

Day/Date: _____

Today I am Grateful for _____

_____

_____

_____

Day/Date: _____

Today I am Grateful for: _____

_____

_____

_____

"The highest tribute to the dead is not grief but gratitude." - Thornton Wilder

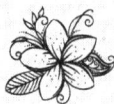

Day/Date: _____

Today I am Grateful for _____

_____

_____

_____

Day/Date: _____

Today I am Grateful for: _____

_____

_____

_____

"Gratitude turns what we can't do into what we can."

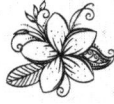

Day/Date: _____

Today I am Grateful for _____

_____

_____

_____

Day/Date: _____

Today I am Grateful for: _____

_____

_____

_____

"Gratitude is the open door to abundance."

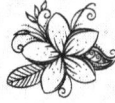

Day/Date: _____

Today I am Grateful for _____

_____

_____

_____

Day/Date: _____

Today I am Grateful for: _____

_____

_____

_____

"Enjoy the little things, for one day you may look back and realize they were the big things." - Robert Brault

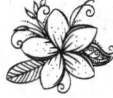

Day/Date: _____

Today I am Grateful for _____

_____

_____

_____

Day/Date: _____

Today I am Grateful for: _____

_____

_____

_____

"Develop an attitude of gratitude, and give thanks for everything that happens to you."
Brian Tracy

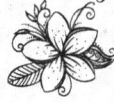

Day/Date: _____

Today I am Grateful for _____

_____

_____

_____

Day/Date: _____

Today I am Grateful for: _____

_____

_____

_____

"Appreciation is a wonderful thing. It makes what is excellent in others belong to us as well." -Voltaire

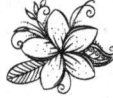

Day/Date: _____

Today I am Grateful for _____

_____

_____

_____

Day/Date: _____

Today I am Grateful for: _____

_____

_____

_____

"Let us be grateful to the people who make us happy." -Marcel Proust

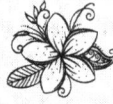

Day/Date: _____

Today I am Grateful for _____

_____

_____

_____

Day/Date: _____

Today I am Grateful for: _____

_____

_____

_____

"Gratitude helps you to grow and expand; gratitude brings joy and laughter into your life." - Eileen Caddy

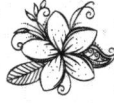

Day/Date: _____

Today I am Grateful for _____

_____

_____

_____

Day/Date: _____

Today I am Grateful for: _____

_____

_____

_____

"Gratitude unlocks the fullness of life." - Melody Beattie

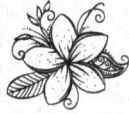

Day/Date: _____

Today I am Grateful for _____

_____

_____

_____

Day/Date: _____

Today I am Grateful for: _____

_____

_____

_____

"Gratitude and attitude are not challenges: they are choices." - Robert Braathe

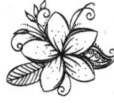

Day/Date: _____

Today I am Grateful for _____

_____

_____

_____

Day/Date: _____

Today I am Grateful for: _____

_____

_____

_____

"Gratitude is the memory of the heart." -Jean Baptiste Massieu

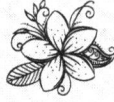

Day/Date: _____

Today I am Grateful for _____

_____

_____

_____

Day/Date: _____

Today I am Grateful for: _____

_____

_____

_____

"Gratitude is a currency that we can mint for ourselves, and spend without fear of bankruptcy." - Fred De Witt Van Amburgh

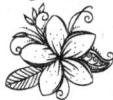

Day/Date: _____

Today I am Grateful for _____

_____

_____

_____

Day/Date: _____

Today I am Grateful for: _____

_____

_____

_____

"Gratitude is a powerful catalyst for happiness." - Amy Collette

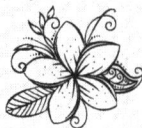

Day/Date: _____

Today I am Grateful for _____

_____

_____

_____

Day/Date: _____

Today I am Grateful for: _____

_____

_____

_____

"The more grateful I am, the more beauty I see." - Mary Davis

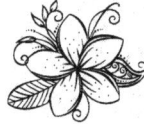

Day/Date: _____

Today I am Grateful for _____

_____

_____

_____

Day/Date: _____

Today I am Grateful for: _____

_____

_____

_____

"Gratitude can transform common days into thanksgivings." -William Arthur Ward

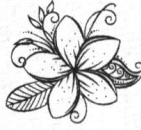

Day/Date: _____

Today I am Grateful for _____

_____

_____

_____

Day/Date: _____

Today I am Grateful for: _____

_____

_____

_____

"Joy is the simplest form of gratitude." - Karl Barth

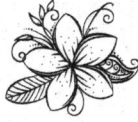

Day/Date: _____

Today I am Grateful for _____

_____

_____

_____

Day/Date: _____

Today I am Grateful for: _____

_____

_____

_____

"The essence of all beautiful art is gratitude." - Friedrich Nietzsche

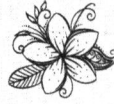

Day/Date: _____

Today I am Grateful for _____

_____

_____

_____

Day/Date: _____

Today I am Grateful for: _____

_____

_____

_____

"Gratitude is the healthiest of all human emotions." - Zig Ziglar

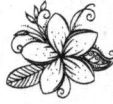

Day/Date: _____

Today I am Grateful for _____

_____

_____

_____

Day/Date: _____

Today I am Grateful for: _____

_____

_____

_____

"The root of joy is gratefulness." - David Steindl-Rast

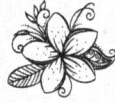

Day/Date: _____

Today I am Grateful for _____

_____

_____

_____

Day/Date: _____

Today I am Grateful for: _____

_____

_____

_____

"Gratitude is the fairest blossom which springs from the soul."
Henry Ward Beecher

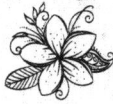

Day/Date: _____

Today I am Grateful for _____

_____

_____

_____

Day/Date: _____

Today I am Grateful for: _____

_____

_____

_____

"When you are grateful, fear disappears and abundance appears." -Anthony Robbins

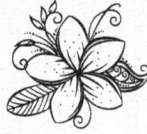

Day/Date: _____

Today I am Grateful for _____

_____

_____

_____

Day/Date: _____

Today I am Grateful for: _____

_____

_____

_____

"Gratitude makes sense of our past, brings peace for today, and creates a vision for tomorrow." - Melody Beattie

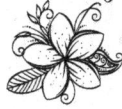

Day/Date: _____

Today I am Grateful for _____

_____

_____

_____

Day/Date: _____

Today I am Grateful for: _____

_____

_____

_____

"Gratitude is not only the greatest of virtues, but the parent of all others." - Cicero

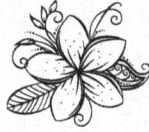

Day/Date: _____

Today I am Grateful for _____

_____

_____

_____

Day/Date: _____

Today I am Grateful for: _____

_____

_____

_____

"Gratitude turns what we have into enough." -Anonymous

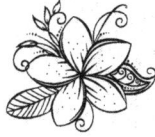

Day/Date: _____

Today I am Grateful for _____

_____

_____

_____

Day/Date: _____

Today I am Grateful for: _____

_____

_____

_____

"Sow kindness, reap gratitude."

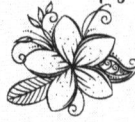

Day/Date: _____

Today I am Grateful for _____

_____

_____

_____

Day/Date: _____

Today I am Grateful for: _____

_____

_____

_____

"Gratitude: life's golden thread."

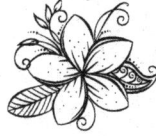

Day/Date: _____

Today I am Grateful for _____

_____

_____

_____

Day/Date: _____

Today I am Grateful for: _____

_____

_____

_____

"Every 'thank you' enriches."

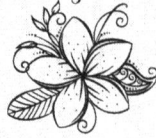

Day/Date: _____

Today I am Grateful for _____

_____

_____

_____

Day/Date: _____

Today I am Grateful for: _____

_____

_____

_____

"Gratitude paints life's canvas."

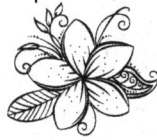

Day/Date: _____

Today I am Grateful for _____

_____

_____

_____

Day/Date: _____

Today I am Grateful for: _____

_____

_____

_____

"Heart full, eyes grateful."

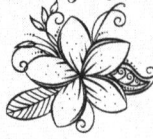

Day/Date: _____

Today I am Grateful for _____

_____

_____

_____

Day/Date: _____

Today I am Grateful for: _____

_____

_____

_____

"Gratitude paints life's canvas."

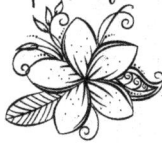

Day/Date: _____

Today I am Grateful for _____

_____

_____

_____

Day/Date: _____

Today I am Grateful for: _____

_____

_____

_____

"Heart full, eyes grateful."

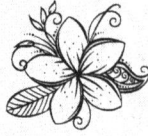

Day/Date: _____

Today I am Grateful for _____

_____

_____

_____

Day/Date: _____

Today I am Grateful for: _____

_____

_____

_____

"Cherish small wonders daily."

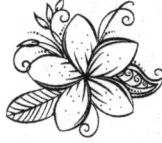

Day/Date: _____

Today I am Grateful for _____

_____

_____

_____

Day/Date: _____

Today I am Grateful for: _____

_____

_____

_____

"Gratitude is soul's music."

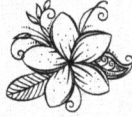

Day/Date: _____

Today I am Grateful for _____

_____

_____

_____

Day/Date: _____

Today I am Grateful for: _____

_____

_____

_____

"Breathe in gratitude, radiate love."

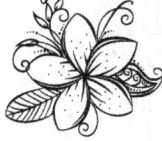

Day/Date: _____

Today I am Grateful for _____

_____

_____

_____

Day/Date: _____

Today I am Grateful for: _____

_____

_____

_____

"Gratitude: the shortest prayer."

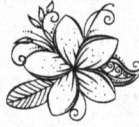

Day/Date: _____

Today I am Grateful for _____

_____

_____

_____

Day/Date: _____

Today I am Grateful for: _____

_____

_____

_____

"Give thanks, gain serenity."

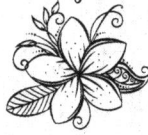

Day/Date: _____

Today I am Grateful for _____

_____

_____

_____

Day/Date: _____

Today I am Grateful for: _____

_____

_____

_____

"Gratitude glows in the humble heart."

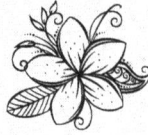

Day/Date: _____

Today I am Grateful for _____

_____

_____

_____

Day/Date: _____

Today I am Grateful for: _____

_____

_____

_____

"Count blessings, multiply joy."

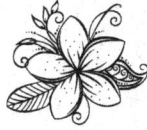

Day/Date: _____

Today I am Grateful for _____

_____

_____

_____

Day/Date: _____

Today I am Grateful for: _____

_____

_____

_____

"Inhale gratitude, exhale contentment."

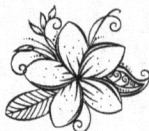

Day/Date: _____

Today I am Grateful for _____

_____

_____

_____

Day/Date: _____

Today I am Grateful for: _____

_____

_____

_____

"Joy is the echo of gratitude in the heart."

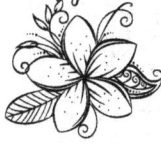

Day/Date: _____

Today I am Grateful for _____

_____

_____

_____

Day/Date: _____

Today I am Grateful for: _____

_____

_____

_____

"Blessed are those who see beauty in small things."

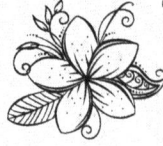

Day/Date: _____

Today I am Grateful for _____

_____

_____

_____

Day/Date: _____

Today I am Grateful for: _____

_____

_____

_____

"Gratitude blossoms where kindness is planted."

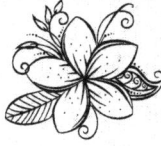

Day/Date: _____

Today I am Grateful for _____

_____

_____

_____

Day/Date: _____

Today I am Grateful for: _____

_____

_____

_____

"Gratitude turns life's melodies harmonious."

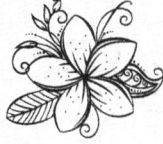

Day/Date: _____

Today I am Grateful for _____

_____

_____

_____

Day/Date: _____

Today I am Grateful for: _____

_____

_____

_____

"Gratitude: the heart's eternal spring."

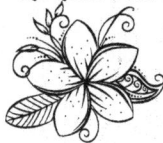

Day/Date: _____

Today I am Grateful for _____

_____

_____

_____

Day/Date: _____

Today I am Grateful for: _____

_____

_____

_____

"In gratitude, every moment flourishes."

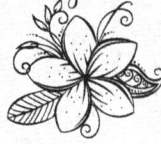

Day/Date: _____

Today I am Grateful for _____

_____

_____

_____

Day/Date: _____

Today I am Grateful for: _____

_____

_____

_____

Gratitude Reflection

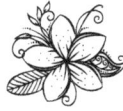

Reflect on the wisdom you've gained over the years. What piece of advice, born from your personal journey, do you feel is essential to pass down to the younger generation, especially young women?

Now that you've spent one year reflecting and showing gratitude, think about a passion or interest you had in your younger years that you haven't pursued lately. How could you rekindle this passion in your current life, and what joy could it bring?

.

Made in the USA
Las Vegas, NV
21 September 2024